JUSTYNA SZYMONIK, MD

How To Get The Most Out Of Your Next Doctor's Visit

A handbook for patients on how to navigate healthcare by getting into your doctor's head.

This book was professionally typeset on Reedsy.
Find out more at reedsy.com

To my parents, Jacek and Jola, for always supporting me during the roughest times of my journey. Kocham was.

To my sisters: Joanna, Magdalena, and Monika, for supporting me in your own ways.

To my med school friends for keeping me sane throughout those 4 years.

To my residency friends, colleagues, and mentors for teaching me everything I know.

And finally, to my patients from the past, present, and future for reminding me of why I got into medicine in the first place.

"It is much more important to know what
sort of a patient has a disease than what
sort of a disease a patient has."

-William Osler

Contents

1

Introduction

If you're reading this book, I just wanted to take a moment to say thank you! Much of what I discuss in this book came from a combination of many discussions I've had with friends, family, co-workers, mentors, (myself), and most importantly, patients. They're the real reason anyone goes into medicine (the ones in it for the long haul, anyway). And throughout my time treating numerous patients, I've learned a few key things. We all have differing experiences growing up, which contribute to us holding different ideas that eventually become our beliefs. When those beliefs become so closely tied to our sense of identity that it becomes who we are, we are significantly more likely to fight back when those ideas are challenged, no matter what they are or how detrimental they may be to us, simply because it becomes a personal fight for our existence. Change rarely happens overnight, especially from reading just one book, so I'm not waiting with bated breath for the world to change once this book is released. Life and experience is ultimately the best teacher for everyone, but the more you can place yourself in someone else's shoes and envision that life experience through their eyes, the more you'll learn about life as a whole. Life is way too short to experience everything yourself, so the next best thing is to check out what others have experienced (be it through books, videos, or whatever media tickles your fancy), and incorporate more of what we like and agree with into our own lives. Too many of us live in our own world and in our own lanes that end up with many of us making the same mistakes over and over again.

Ultimately, what I ask of you, the reader is to evaluate your own experience in the healthcare system (the good, the bad, and the ugly) and then revisit it through your medical provider's eyes. If you have no idea how to do that, this book should be a good first step. Before I went into medicine, I had virtually no experience or knowledge of the field, so the goal of this book is to take you through my journey and hopefully leave you all a little more knowledgeable about how the US healthcare system actually works, and with a lot more understanding of what your doctor's job actually entails. This is your exclusive sneak peek behind the curtain, all the things I'd tell you if you were family or a close friend. This is some of what I and my fellow colleagues paid over $200K in medical school tuition to learn. With that being said, sit back, grab your cozy beverage of choice, and let's dive in together.

*Disclaimer: Even though I am a doctor, I am not your doctor. This book is not meant to guide medical treatment; it only serves to provide general teaching points. Do not discontinue your medications or change your course of treatment without consulting **your** physician or other healthcare provider.

2

The Chief Complaint: "OK… So What Hurts the Most?"

Many people love putting off going to the doctor. It seems to be one of those universal truths, along with putting off seeing the dentist and doing our taxes. Many times, we end up living reactively and only address those issues when we have external factors pushing on us (toothaches, Tax Day, etc). So when that one concern of ours becomes more than an everyday ache, we finally plan that whole day excursion to go to the doctor's office. However, because we are all fans of efficiency, we might as well ask the doctor about that one spot on our arm, right?

And is it normal for my ears to ring randomly throughout the day? And my grandma's sister had breast cancer, does that mean I need a mammogram? As our mind buzzes with more and more questions, we also sense a growing frustration with the doctor as our appointment time passes. "What's the big idea… I got here 15 minutes early and the doctor **still** isn't here?! This is ridiculous!"

Imagine this:

3

You work an office job in a high-rise in a major city. You've got a big meeting planned for today with some clients first thing in the morning. You've prepared the night before by reviewing their files and anticipating their needs. You come to work a little early to make sure everything's in place. Your secretary blocked off an hour in your schedule for the encounter, ensuring time to build rapport, go through your presentation, and answer any lingering questions at the end, as well as ensuring a buffer before your next meeting.

Now, instead of the high-rise in the big city, imagine you're in a small, 2-story building. Instead of donning a business jacket, you grab a white coat. Instead of carrying a briefcase, you're equipped with your stethoscope. And instead of the comfortable, hour-long meetings with clients, you have 20 of them back-to-back, with each lasting a brief 15 minutes before someone pops into your room to alert you that your next client (or rather, patient) is already waiting with their concerns.

This becomes the everyday struggle that many doctors face, especially those in primary care. The system is set up (notably <u>not</u> by physicians) so that each appointment typically takes up a time slot lasting 15 minutes (or in some cases, 30 minutes for the initial visit), and the doctor gets to use whatever is left of that time slot after the intake and vitals are completed. Although the people we see are complicated beings, each with their own experiences, fears, and beliefs, the system addresses this by having us reduce the people we see to just **one** complaint at the visit. So you may have heard your doctor ask you, "What's going on today?" but really what they're asking is more along the lines of, "So what's your most concerning issue that actually brought you in today?" We all have many concerns hounding us daily, but this visit becomes a place where we can devote our energy and resources to getting to the bottom of at least one of them.

I've heard many people scoff at this (including my own family) and say things like, "Oh, they just want me to keep making appointments to get as much money out of me as possible." This can be frustrating on a number of levels, but perhaps the biggest reason this doesn't sit well with most medical providers is that it assumes we care more about your wallet than your health, which for most is the farthest thing from the truth. The other practical reason we try not to book each patient more than they actually need to be seen is because the biggest resource that most doctors are lacking is that of time. We have so much on our plate that if we don't need to see you, we don't actually *want* to see you (apart from the occasional run-in at the local grocery store). Most of us care about our patients so much that we plan our follow-up visits so that we can decrease the chance of the dreaded "surprise" visit. Just like with your car, if you get your oil changed when it's due instead of waiting until there's a problem, it might cost a little more money upfront, but overall, you'll be saving hundreds (if not thousands) of dollars down the road.

So that's what our visit ends up being centered on; something we like to call the *Chief Complaint* which, just like it sounds, is the most important concern. We'll talk more about how that gets evaluated in the next chapter, but it's important to keep it in mind as this marks the beginning of the medical investigation. All of the questions, labs, images, and potential specialists that follow are all in response to that initial clue. In some cases, it may start out as one thing and turn into something else. For instance, if you walk in with toe pain, but it turns out that you've also been having chest pain on and off for several weeks, then that becomes the new *Chief Complaint* since ruling out a heart attack falls higher on our priority list than an achy toe.

What should your doctor be doing, or what exactly is their role here?

There is a technique we use called "Agenda Setting" that helps us organize your concerns and develop a plan. Just like you might list all of the tasks you have to take care of in a to-do list and schedule time to do them, this technique allows for a doctor to list all of the patient's concerns, and then develop a plan to address them. It should look something like asking the following questions:

1. What brought you in today?
2. Any other concerns?
3. OK, any *other* concerns?
4. Alright, it sounds like [X], [Y], and [Z] are bothering you today. We won't have enough time to adequately address all of these concerns today; are you OK if we address [insert most concerning complaint] today, and then we can plan to follow up and address the other ones another time?

Now, this might look simple, but I can assure you that it's much easier said than done. When I was first starting as a resident, this conversation was either driven by A) my initial instinct to dive right into the first concern that popped up in conversation, or B) by the patient's assertiveness to discuss whatever they wanted. However, we would then get to the dilemma of arriving at the end of the visit, getting ready to see the next patient, only to be ambushed by a, "By the way doc, I've been having bloody diarrhea for some time…" So, if you've still been wondering why doctors run late to their appointments so frequently, sometimes it's because we've got to be flexible enough to make sure that those important comments are appropriately addressed.

So, my fellow reader, what do you do now? What is your call to action?

The next time you go to the doctor, keep this in mind. When they ask you questions about your concern, try to keep it focused on the complaint at hand, unless it otherwise shifts or you truly have something else you are more worried about. If you have multiple concerns, it's a great idea to come prepared with a written list! And if your doctor didn't ask you the questions above to list them all out, start out the visit by saying, "I have several concerns today. Is it OK if we make a plan to check them out?" If the doctor hasn't done so already, this primes the conversation to address what needs to be addressed in a timely manner for both parties. It allows for reasonable expectations, which can completely shift our perception (and satisfaction) of the visit. Knowing what can and can't be done in a certain amount of time allows us to focus our attention on addressing the task at hand. By having reasonable expectations ahead of time, we aren't worried about the unreasonable things we otherwise might've been worried about.

Health care is not meant to be a one-time thing. It is a long-term investment into one of our most valuable investments, the biological vehicle we carry throughout our entire lives, our bodies. The more we can take ownership of our health, the more of it we realize we can control, and the more potential we have to feel empowered and cherish it!

3

The Art of the History

One of the worst medical dramas to date (at least in terms of accuracy) has got to be *House MD*. Not only do they have the same doctors perform every single procedure, regularly break into the homes of their patients, and order (often dangerous) treatments before the simpler and more reasonable diagnostic testing, they never get the full story! Most people think doctors figure out what's happened to a patient through whatever labs and imaging they order through the hospital. However, at the start of medical school we're taught that the diagnosis can be made with just the medical history alone roughly 80% of the time! That's right, the descriptors you use are enough to guide us (mostly) to the right answer. They point us in the direction of what tests to order and what your prognosis might look like.

So, for example, the chest pain that is described as *pressure* vs *stabbing* vs *tearing* make us think of 3 wildly different scenarios, which we further distinguish between while asking more questions. Just like seeing darker clouds in the sky might increase the chance of rain that day (but not guarantee it), the presence (or absence) of certain features make certain diagnoses more (or less) likely to be the culprit.

History of Present Illness (HPI):

So, to cover all of our bases, we like to use acronyms like OLD CARTS. Fun, right?!

It covers all the basic questions that your doctor should be asking you:

O - Onset: When did the pain start?

L - Location: Where is it located?

D - Duration: How long has it been going on?

C - Character: How would you describe the pain?

A - Alleviating/Aggravating: What seems to make it better or worse?

R - Radiation: Does the pain seem to move to another location?

T - Temporal: Do you find that your pain seems to change depending on the time of day, or depending on what you're doing?

S - Severity: How bad is the pain? (On a scale from 1–10)

Sometimes we don't go through every single one of these questions (it might not be very helpful to ask where in someone's body their depression is located), but it gives us a great place to start when gathering the history. In fact, these are the questions we have to answer for every concern you have when we write up our patient notes for billing and insurance! And remember when we said that we can only really address one complaint at a time? This is one of the reasons why—we have to run through this list of questions for every concern that you bring us. However, if you're experiencing other symptoms that appear to be related to your initial complaint, this brings us to the next section, which we'll discuss below.

Review of Systems (ROS):

To summarize so far, what I've just covered is what we like to call the *HPI* or *History of Present Illness*. It contains your story as it relates to the questions listed above. It typically also contains a list of associated symptoms called the *ROS* or *Review of Systems*. Although some symptoms can show up on their own, oftentimes they show up with a group of closely related symptoms that together make up a syndrome. When most people hear "syndrome", they may initially think of something like "Down syndrome", which is one example of the term. It's defined as having a partial or complete additional copy of chromosome 21 and is associated with a group of physical features that typically occur together including a flattened face, almond-shaped eyes, and shorter neck to name a few. Now consider a heart attack — some of the common, textbook symptoms commonly seen include chest pain/pressure, nausea, sweating, and pain radiating to the left arm and/or jaw to name a few. This collection of symptoms could also technically be considered a syndrome because they all have been proven to occur together and are likely caused by the same thing. However, we don't go around saying someone has a "heart attack syndrome" because the presentation of a heart attack has much more variability in the real world and in different populations (especially men vs women — yet another reason why we leave diagnosing up to the professionals). But the premise here is similar: we have several theories as to what could be going on, and we expect to see certain symptoms with certain disease states. So what your doctor should do at this stage is to ask about any other (recent) symptoms that you've experienced, and they'll do so by organ systems. Expect more detailed questions about the organ system of concern, and more general questions to cover the bases.

An example of a very basic review of systems (again, asking about **recent** symptoms) should look something like this:

General: Any fevers, chills, night sweats? Any unexplained weight loss?
   HEENT (Head, Ears, Eyes, Nose, Throat)
   Head: Any headaches?
   Eyes: Any vision changes or eye pain?
   Ears: Any hearing loss or ear pain?
   Nose: Any nose bleeds or discharge?
   Cardiovascular: Any chest pain or heart palpitations?
   Pulmonary: Any shortness of breath, with movement or at rest?
   Gastrointestinal: Any nausea, vomiting, diarrhea/constipation?
   MSK (Musculoskeletal): Any muscle aches or joint pains?
   Skin: Any rashes?
   Genitourinary: Any burning with urination? Any discharge?
   Heme/Lymphatics: Any easy bleeding/bruising, or any issues with
swelling in your arms/legs?
   Neurological: Any numbness or weakness? Any recent loss of
consciousness?
   Psychological: Any mood changes? Any visual/auditory hallucina-
tions?

The symptoms that we expect to be present in a given situation, if
present, are called *pertinent positives;* likewise, the symptoms that we may
expect to be present (but are not) are referred to as *pertinent negatives*.
These findings, along with the other features we discussed under **HPI**,
together increase or decrease the likelihood of you having a certain
diagnosis, or what we like to refer to as the *pretest probability*. It might
sound complicated, but it simply refers to how certain we are that you
may have a certain diagnosis before checking any tests.

Past Medical History:

The last main component of history taking is, well, recording your medical history! This is where we get to address what's happening to you, presently, in the context of what's happened to you before. Someone who's having chest pain for the very first time with no other medical history is very different from the person who's having chest pain with a history of multiple heart attacks, coronary stent placements, and a quadruple bypass. In my personal experience, it appears to be one of the more neglected sides of medicine, with the potential to have some egregious consequences. I've had the opportunity to accompany my family members to their doctors multiple times during my training and found myself having to supplement their history by volunteering critical pieces of information that the doctor should have asked for. Whether they were pressed for time or just forgot, it doesn't actually matter- doctors are human, are therefore not perfect, and are likely to miss something at some point. By writing about it here, I want to compel you, as the reader, to share in the burden that is your health. By knowing what to expect, you can help verify that we as your doctor understand the situation completely.

To paint the initial picture, the histories they should go through with you, in no particular order, should look something like this:

Past Medical History:

- What medical conditions do you have that you see a doctor for?
- Have you had to see a specialist before? What was that for?
- Have you ever been hospitalized? What for?

Current Medications:

- What prescription medications do you take? What are the doses?

- Do you take them as instructed? If not, why?
- What supplements do take?

Allergies:

- Do you have any adverse reactions to any medications or materials (i.e. latex)? If so, what is the reaction? (rash, trouble breathing, nausea, etc)

Surgical History:

- Have you had any surgeries in the past? What were they, what were they done for, and when were they done? Were there any complications?

Social History:

- <u>Social connections</u>: (age dependent) Are you single/married? What is your highest level of education? If employed, what do you do for work? Are you concerned about finances? Do you have a supportive group of family/friends nearby? Do you have trouble connecting with people?
- <u>Lifestyle</u>:

1. Diet: What does your current diet look like? Do you have any questions or concerns about your current diet?
2. Exercising: Are you currently exercising? Are you getting at least 150 minutes of moderate-intensity exercise per week? Are you incorporating weightlifting? Do you engage in yoga or other stretching/mobility/flexibility practices regularly? If you aren't currently exercising, what are the barriers that are preventing you

from doing so?

3. Sleep: How is your sleep? Do you have problems with going to sleep, staying asleep, or waking up rested? Do you require sleeping aids to sleep?

4. Stress: Do you have any significant stressors in your life? How do you usually cope? Do you regularly practice gratitude, either verbally and/or through journaling? How do you spend a typical day? What hobbies do you enjoy? Have you been able to engage in your hobbies recently?

- Tobacco: Do you smoke tobacco currently or in the past? How many packs a day, and for how many years? Do you vape? How frequently?

- Illicit/Recreational Drug Use: Do you use any illicit drugs or medications not prescribed for you? How often, and when was the last use? Have you ever experienced withdrawals? Have you been to a rehab center? Do you have a support group to lean on as needed?

- Alcohol: Do you drink alcohol currently or in the past? How often/regularly? How many drinks per week, and what kind of alcohol is it? Have you ever had issues with withdrawal or seizures related to alcohol use? Have you ever been hospitalized for alcohol use?

- Sexual: Are you sexually active? Is it oral, anal, vaginal, or a combination? With men, women, or both? How many different partners have you had in the last year? Do you use protection (i.e. condoms, birth control, IUD)? Have you and your partner(s) received the Gardasil vaccines?

- Trauma: Have you experienced physical/emotional/verbal/sexual abuse, or witnessed it firsthand? Do you currently feel safe at home and with your current relationships? Do you have trustworthy people you can reach out to if needed?

Family History:

- Do your biological parents, grandparents, aunts/uncles or siblings have any medical conditions that they see a doctor for? If they've passed, what did they pass from, and at what age?
- Any history of any cancers in the family (siblings, parents, grandparents)? If so, at what age were they diagnosed?

(When in the hospital) Code Status:

- (Full Code) Would you like us to perform all life-saving measures to prolong your life? If your heart were to stop beating, would you like us to perform chest compressions, knowing that you may experience broken ribs as a result? And if you were to stop breathing, would you like us to intubate you and have you on the ventilator?

It's important for you to personally be able to answer all of these questions. You will not get asked them all at the same time, but that doesn't mean it shouldn't be addressed. And the other big note here is to be as honest as possible! I know that in the social history section, for example, the questions can get a little dicey, but I can promise you that we won't judge you for your answers. We have a reason for every question we ask you, and if it makes you feel better, you can always ask us for that reason.

So what is the takeaway for you here?

1. **Knowledge is power!** _Take some time going through all the questions listed here._ If you don't have anything bothering you at this time, make sure that you're able to go through all of the past medical history questions to make sure there isn't anything alarming. If you suddenly show up in the office with bloody diarrhea in your 30s, and you found out last week that your uncle and grandfather both had colon cancer in their 40s, that will immediately get our attention and adjust our recommendations. If you have any concerns about any of your answers to these questions, then that could be a great thing to talk to your doctor about.

2. **Be honest.** Help us help you! As I mentioned above, some people may want to leave out some details like drug use, but it's extremely important for us to know as much as we can about the situation. Simply put, different drugs have different effects, and we want to know what to expect and plan for appropriate treatment. We do have tests that can check for a variety of drugs, but if you tell us first then we can start those treatments right away, and make sure we won't give you anything to make your condition worse. Some people may worry about us telling their family or the police, but in most cases, HIPAA laws prevent us from doing so.

3. **Stay on topic.** When giving your story to the healthcare provider in the clinic/hospital, try to make sure that your story addresses all the questions they ask as much as possible. If your provider didn't ask you one of these questions, and it's applicable to you and to the concern at hand, consider volunteering that information! Or, if you prefer for the provider to take the lead and ask you all the relevant questions, do your best to be as direct as possible. I've heard time and time again from family and friends, justifying their "word vomit" as "Well I don't know what information will actually help the doctor, so I'll just tell them everything that runs across my mind." I know everyone here means well, but if you're the 7th

person to tell me about your cousin's stepdad's mother's childhood asthma, and I've got 4 more patients waiting to be seen, then you could see how we could get stressed for time.

4. **Get involved!** Be an active member in taking care of your health. If you have certain suspicions, for whatever reason, let us know! The best doctors will leave space for you to contribute your thoughts with a question like, ***"What do you think is going on?"*** This isn't us asking you to do our job for us, but rather getting a pulse on your insight. Although we know the medicine, you're the one who knows your body the best, and therefore knows when something's not right. It's also a great time for us to address any concerns you might have at the time. If you just read an article on colon cancer and then noticed a little blood in your stool, even if it's from something else, that's still a worthwhile discussion to have with your doctor. We can talk about risk factors, signs to look out for, and reasons why or why not it applies to your case.

5. **Reflect**. As I mentioned before, just because your doctor doesn't mention something doesn't mean it's not important. Especially those in the lifestyle subsection— I can guarantee that 98% of people have never been asked those questions directly unless they were specifically seeing a board-certified lifestyle medicine doctor (which yes, may be a surprise to many, but they do in fact exist). However, some people will never stop to consider these factors unless they're specifically asked about them! And it's specifically those factors that, if addressed early enough, oftentimes may prevent (or at least improve) other medical complications and conditions. That's why I did my best to be as thorough with these questions as possible so that they can serve as a good starting point for those who truly want to live their healthiest lives, whether it be for themselves or their family. My recommendation here is to answer these questions (especially those in the lifestyle subsection)

like a journaling prompt and get into them as much as you can for your own sake. However, if you find yourself getting stuck, your provider is an excellent resource to go to for additional help and information! For example, if you've always wondered about the "ideal diet", your provider is a great first stop! At the very least, they can always point you in the right direction (i.e. refer you to a dietitian, support group, etc).

At this point, your doctor should be coming up with a list of potential causes for your condition. The idea is that, as we progress through the visit, the list will get smaller and smaller. So, feel free to ask your doctor, "What do you think it could be?" but only if you're comfortable getting back some variation of, "I'm not sure yet."

How do we become more sure? Let's keep going!

4

Let's Get (a) Physical (Exam)

At this point in the visit, in most cases, your doctor should have a pretty good idea of what's going on. All of the information we've acquired up to this point, although considered subjective since it's only been given through you and your experience, has likely narrowed down the list of possibilities to just a few. This is where we start to introduce objective information, or information that is not influenced by the feelings, opinions, or experiences of any one person. In the same way that a court will listen to eyewitness testimony, but still rely on physical evidence before ultimately deciding on a verdict, your doctor will use a combination of your story and the objective evidence they collect to make a final say on your diagnosis.

The exact exam that a doctor might give you might vary wildly based on your complaint. There are many things we can test for, but just because we can test for them doesn't mean we do. The only exception might be if a medical student is learning how to perform the maneuvers for their learning. If you're just getting a regular physical during a wellness visit, then your doctor might perform a series of regular examinations to get a good baseline for how you are. Otherwise, if you come in for

19

a particular concern, like difficulty breathing, then you can bet that your doctor will be spending more time listening to your lungs than examining your ankles or your elbows.

All exams actually start with your vitals, which should already be available for us to examine by the time we see you. As the name suggests, your vitals are vital for us to know! They can give us a snapshot of how healthy or sick you are at any given point. Whatever medical professional sees you first, whether it's in the hospital or clinic, be it EMS, nurses, or medical assistants, they are all trained to take this "snapshot" so we can monitor your status. The components of your vitals they're specifically measuring typically include your temperature, pulse (heart rate), blood pressure, respiratory rate (measured in the number of breaths per minute), and oxygen saturation levels. If any of these are severely out of range, that alone can be enough to send you to the hospital (if you're not already there) or to move you to a more critical floor (if you are).

For the actual exam, your doctor will examine you through a systems-based approach, similar to the ROS we mentioned in the last chapter. However, instead of addressing a list of subjective questions (did you feel XYZ?), it becomes a list of findings that the doctor checked for and either discovered or did not discover during their exam. A basic general exam (with normal results) would look something like this:

General: No acute distress, well-appearing.
  HEENT (Head, Ears, Eyes, Nose, Throat)
  Head: Atraumatic, normocephalic.
  Eyes: EOMI (extra-ocular movements intact).
  Ears: Ear canals patent, Tympanic membranes intact.
  Nose: No septal deviation present, Normal-appearing nasal

turbinates.

Cardiovascular: RRR (regular rate and rhythm).

Pulmonary: CTAB (clear to auscultation bilaterally), Equal chest wall expansion.

Gastrointestinal: Soft, Non-tender to palpation, Non-distended in all quadrants, Normal bowel sounds.

MSK (Musculoskeletal): Full ROM (range of motion), No joint effusion or swelling.

Integumentary (Skin): Warm, No rashes or lesions.

Genitourinary: No flank pain bilaterally.

Endocrine: No palpable thyroid nodules appreciated.

Lymphatics: No palpable cervical, axillary, or femoral lymph nodes bilaterally.

Neurological: CN (cranial nerves) II-XII intact, Strength 5/5 in bilateral upper and lower extremities, Sensation intact.

Psychological: Normal mood and affect, Linear speech.

If you couldn't understand a good portion of the text above, that's OK- it's part of the "doctor speak" that we learn in medical school that helps us convey very particular ideas to one another. The point I'm trying to make is how we address all these systems (to varying degrees) every time we examine you, even if you might not realize it.

In most scenarios, when you are alert enough to have a conversation with us, we are able to use our physical exam findings to supplement the information we've been given thus far. However, if you're brought in by the paramedics because you were found unconscious and alone, and no one really knows what happened, then the physical exam suddenly carries much more weight. Your vitals and physical exam become the basis for our evaluation, at least until we're able to contact someone who might be able to give us more information.

Inconsistencies

Another example of the importance of the physical exam comes whenever there's a question of physical abuse. I once had a mother bring her child in with a burn mark on his torso, telling me that there was an accident in the kitchen where he pulled a cup of hot water off the counter, and accidentally spilled some on himself. Although the story seemed plausible, as the child was old enough to walk without support, young enough to cause unknowing trouble to himself, and didn't seem fearful of anyone, I still wanted to do my due diligence and consult with my attending doctors at the time to verify that the pattern of the markings was consistent with an accident. They agreed with my assessment, and we had the mother and patient follow up closely to make sure our burn care recommendations were working. In the end, it worked out well because they showed up to the follow-up appointments, no new injuries were found, and the patient was healing nicely (all of which support accidental over intentional injury). With children or the elderly, where we might not always be able to get a reliable history from the patient themselves, the physical exam can play a larger role than it would otherwise. If we're given one story, and the exam findings don't reasonably match it, that can raise a red flag for us.

There are times when someone describes an issue (like pain) where the doctor examines them and they can't find anything wrong, so they end up dismissing the complaint. This is one of the biggest misconceptions about medicine, and something that many doctors have been terrible about communicating, so I'd like to try to clear the air as best as I can. **Just because your physical exam was normal, doesn't mean that there's nothing wrong!** It just means that some of the things we can check for on an exam didn't show up as abnormal. That means that whatever is ailing you is beyond our ability to check for it at this point in time. **The doctors who don't believe that you're telling the truth simply because they can't find the cause for your symptoms are the ones you need to run from.** A doctor who chooses not to believe you and your story will likely not be your best advocate throughout your healthcare journey. If possible, keep looking for a doctor who will be honest, advocate for you, and address your concerns instead of dismissing them. Your doctor doesn't have to know all the right answers to be the best, they just have to commit their best to discovering the answer with you.

5

Labs and Imaging: Treating the Numbers vs Treating the Patient

Whenever my mother brought me and my siblings to the doctor's office for our yearly physicals growing up, we would almost always get our blood drawn. We were generally healthy kids, so usually our lab work was largely normal. A lower Vitamin D level here, lower hemoglobin there, it wasn't anything we couldn't fix with sunlight and an iron-rich diet. Then, once I was in college, I had a new abnormality pop up— a slightly elevated bilirubin. I had no idea what it meant at the time, and since I felt fine, it didn't bother me; however, it did make me curious. When I showed it to my mother, who had previously worked as a nurse years ago, her anxiety skyrocketed. At that time, all she remembered was that bilirubin was associated with the liver, which led her to jump to all sorts of conclusions, namely accusing me of excessive drinking. Knowing that that couldn't be the case, reflecting on how infrequently and minimally I engaged with drinking, I decided to reach back out to my doctor to learn more. She explained that she suspected it could be something called, "Gilbert's syndrome", but decided to send me to see a gastroenterologist so he could verify. Sure enough, weeks later I met with the GI doctor,

24

who drew more blood and had me come back a few weeks later, after speaking with a hepatologist (liver specialist) to tell me that it was in fact, Gilbert's syndrome. For those of you reading this who don't know what Gilbert's syndrome is, all you have to know is that it doesn't mean much. Technically, it's a condition where the liver is a little less efficient than average at processing and breaking down bilirubin, but realistically it means nothing. Apart from maybe experiencing a little jaundice in times of excessive fasting or stress, it has no symptoms, and the prognosis isn't different from anyone else.

So what's the takeaway here?

Sometimes the stress of a potential harm is the biggest harm there is. I could have lived the rest of my life not knowing about this small abnormality and it wouldn't have changed my life in the slightest. My example wasn't the most alarming, but the premise is the same with anyone trying the "just to make sure" testing. Instead of a small variation in a lab value, it could be a small spot found on someone's lung during a CT scan that someone really insisted on getting (commonly termed an "incidental finding"). Then, because everyone's first concern with new spots on imaging is potential cancer, the next step is to wait and see if it gets any bigger, or in some cases, undergo an invasive biopsy. Then, 6 months later, you get a repeat scan just to find out that it's the same size. Then you get yearly scans, and every year it's the same size. When patients who have tons of money, power, and influence try to persuade their doctor to order every test under the sun, this is exactly what they may fall victim to.

Although the process of phlebotomy and bloodletting has been around since ancient times, the labs and imaging of today are great tools that have really only been around recently. The first x-rays were observed in the 1890s, while CT and MRI machines made their debut in the public eye in the 1970s. While they have their place, many have mistaken their purpose.

The truth is, every lab and imaging study has to be ordered with a specific purpose in mind. Their main job is to either support or refute our hypotheses about what may be going on with a patient. If someone is having trouble breathing, we might order a chest x-ray if we suspect they could have pneumonia. However, just because someone has a complaint like difficulty breathing doesn't mean we need to jump to that chest x-ray if it is more likely explained by something else. For example, if someone's having difficulty moving air through their lungs, but they've run out of their inhaler for their asthma and present with wheezing on their physical exam, then we might try a breathing treatment to address the asthma and see if it improves before blindly ordering a chest x-ray.

In general, we tend to order tests for these reasons:

1. Screening (certain populations)
2. Aid in confirming/rejecting a suspected diagnosis
3. Monitor status/prognosis

Screening guidelines are in place because there's a big enough collection of data to suggest that some people, depending on their age or other lifestyle factors, would have more benefit than risk from checking certain tests. A low-dose CT scan in someone who has a significant smoking history is a reasonable screening test once they reach a certain age, but not in someone who doesn't smoke or has other risk factors. Others, like colonoscopies, are generally recommended for everyone over a certain age, regardless of other risk factors. In this case, it's because we've noticed the increase in the prevalence of colon cancer as people get older, and the process for checking and removing suspicious polyps is pretty effective since they can be removed as soon as they're spotted.

So before placing any orders for any tests, your doctor should be ready to answer these questions:

1. What are we expecting to see?
2. What are we going to do about it?

If we can't give a definitive answer to those questions, then we likely don't need to order any tests. In some rare cases, if your doctor has no idea what's going on, they may take the "shotgun" approach to give them some clues, but this is generally avoided and frowned upon. Labs without the context of the patient are just numbers. A hemoglobin of 12 in one patient who's well and active is wildly different than that same hemoglobin of 12 in someone who's actively and profusely bleeding with a previously recorded hemoglobin of 15 from the day prior. Even though it's the same lab value for both patients, the management is wildly different because of the context.

So **don't be afraid to take the extra time and ask your doctor** about your tests! Not only what they mean, but why they ordered it. If they don't take the time to explain to you why they're checking a certain test, especially after you asked them, then you should reconsider having them as your provider. Our job is not only to diagnose and treat you, but to empower you with medical literacy about your own health so that no matter where you go, you'll be able to advocate for yourself even if the people around you won't. After all, the original word *doctor* in Latin translates to "teacher", which means that teaching you about your health is not just a fun perk of our job, but truly a core tenet of it.

6

Diagnosis: "So What's Wrong with Me?"

One of the main reasons you likely made that first trip to the doctor is to answer the question, "So why am I actually sick?". You might have some inklings based on your personal experience (i.e. you feel similar to that one time you had the flu, so maybe it's the flu again?), but it can be just as harmful as it is helpful depending on the context. This is why a doctor's first job is usually diagnosing the problem (assuming you're not actively dying, in which case we'll start supportive treatment before we get the whole story). Having a label for your condition is nice, but the more important information we're looking for is the suspected course and prognosis that's associated with the label. If your throat is sore from a simple upper respiratory infection (usually caused by a virus), we know from a large collection of data/evidence that your symptoms should reliably subside after a few days to weeks and that we aren't suspecting any long-term consequences. However, if your throat is sore because you have an active strep infection, then we'll treat that with an antibiotic, but not for the reason you might think. Although antibiotics have been shown to reduce the length of time you experience symptoms slightly, most people will actually clear these infections on their own. The main benefit of giving antibiotics to these patients is actually to reduce the risk of developing a future complication known as Rheumatic Fever in the future, which can then affect your heart valves. You aren't expected to know all of this nuance, of course, but this is simply to illustrate that the problems in front of us aren't always straightforward ones.

"...Think Horses not Zebras"

The whole process of diagnosing a patient starts the moment we hear about your Chief Complaint. Immediately we begin forming a list called a *Differential Diagnosis*, or a list of possible diagnoses that could be causing your symptoms. It typically starts off extremely broad and then becomes narrowed as we collect more and more information. Sometimes potential diagnoses can be completely taken off the list, and other times they're just moved down and labeled "less likely at this time".

This is one example where we can see the art of medicine take place— no two doctors will come up with exactly the same list. If you've ever wondered why "getting a second opinion" can be helpful, it's precisely for this reason. Fresh eyes will consider new options through their own brainstorming session. Just as asking 2 people to list the first 10 pieces of fruit that come to mind may share some common fruits (apples, bananas, oranges), chances are that there will be some variability throughout each person's list as it goes on.

The medical variation of trying to list the most common culprits can be seen through the phrase "If you hear hoofbeats…think horses, not zebras!" This refers to thinking about the most common or likely causes for a certain symptom first. Sure, in medical school we learned about the "exotic" pathologies like the "pheochromocytoma" (aka a tumor of the adrenal glands) in cases of high blood pressure, and in certain cases, we want to make sure that they end up on our differential. However, if there are much likelier options that we haven't considered or addressed beforehand, then we're doing you a disservice by not looking at those first. The reason why certain shows like *House MD* take off is because they like to live in a world where all of the answers are "zebras". Why? Well, it's not nearly as exciting to see someone's blood pressure elevated as a result of obesity as it is to see blood pressure elevated from a rare, adrenaline-secreting tumor.

Knowing vs Not Knowing vs Knowing What It's Not

In a perfect world, your doctor would always know exactly what's going on and also know exactly what to do to treat it. However, life tends to get a little more complicated. Sometimes important pieces of the history might be missing, or you might have an uncommon presentation of your illness, or you might actually have one of the rare diseases that get shown on medical shows like *House MD*, in which case your doctor likely won't even know how to check for it. So, what the game of diagnosis comes down to is figuring out "Do we know what's going on, and with what certainty?" as well as "Can we at least rule certain disease states out?".

"Knowing" a certain diagnosis, as I've outlined throughout this book, is a process. It starts with getting a good idea of what's going on (the history), then confirming or denying our suspicions with our findings (physical exam, lab/imaging results). By the end, if we're lucky, we have a good idea of what's going on, one possible diagnosis that is more likely than the rest. However, when the evidence doesn't line up as neatly for whatever reason, we might not be able to decide on a particular diagnosis with the same level of certainty each time. However, in our quest to find out what the diagnosis could be, we oftentimes will rule out what it likely isn't, and that can be just as important (if not more important) in many cases. If you go to the emergency room for chest pain, you will undergo some form of what many of us call a "Chest pain rule-out". Basically, that just refers to ruling out a heart attack, which includes monitoring labs like Troponin (which measures specific proteins found in the heart muscle) as well as an EKG. If your test results come back normal, but you're still experiencing chest pain, then our work is not done but we have made progress. Being able to say "At least we know you're not having a heart attack" is huge! Not that there aren't other dangerous causes of chest pain, which depending on certain parts of your history can prompt us to pursue other imaging and labs, but it's one of the major causes of mortality, especially in the US, so ruling it out cannot be undersold.

"Don't be Heuri-sterical"

Heuristics. Most people don't realize it, but it's likely the most common cause of most people's frustration with their individual doctors outside of the logistics of healthcare. Most of the horror stories that people will share with each other through forums on the internet are born as a result of it.

And yet we can't escape it.

A heuristic can broadly be understood as a problem-solving method that involves a "cognitive shortcut". It's how we come to the decisions that we make. In the context of medicine, it's usually referring to how we make our diagnosis.

Broadly speaking, it can be divided into 2 groups, Analytical and Intuitive, each with their own pros and cons. I'll just be brushing the surface as this is a large enough topic to write a separate book on.

Analytical reasoning is how most people start off learning. It involves deliberate deduction and consideration of the evidence presented, much like a lawyer would use to put together her case. It is more time-intensive and uses more cognitive resources, but in the end, you have a road map that explains how you arrived at a certain conclusion, and others can easily follow along.

Intuitive reasoning is typically seen in more experienced practitioners. Once someone gains more and more experience, they begin to notice certain patterns presented before them, sometimes consciously, other times unconsciously. You arrive at an answer much quicker than you would following the analytical route and therefore use fewer cognitive resources, but the accuracy of your answer may be called into question because the path you've taken to get there oftentimes isn't as clear. It doesn't necessarily mean that the answer you arrive at is wrong (in fact, many rely on this method because of how many times they got the answer right!), but you may not have all the evidence you need to verify that it's correct. And just like the name suggests, it relies on one's intuition, which can be thought of as "knowing without knowing why". It has its benefits, like knowing what to do if someone is crashing before you, or it might give you inspiration for tackling a problem with a different approach if you're stuck, but it has the potential for many problems.

So knowing this, which one would you choose, or want your doctor to choose? Analytical, right?

Well, it turns out that the human brain will do almost anything to reduce its workload. That's right, the default we all have, if we have the experience to back it up, will be Intuitive reasoning, regardless of how we feel about that consciously. Despite the benefit of Analytical reasoning, our brains will try to convince us that it's not worth pursuing in every single case, and in some cases, that might even prove to be correct if we end up coming to the correct conclusion.

What does this look like in medicine? The following are examples of the types of errors we see in cognitive biases, or specifically the mental shortcuts we take when dealing with objective information:

1. *Anchoring bias*: This refers to a phenomenon where a clinician will prematurely decide (or "anchor") on a diagnosis based on some preliminary evidence, usually in the context of their personal experience. If a physician just saw 4 patients back-to-back with chest pain, and the first 3 were found to have heart attacks, then that physician might prematurely jump to the conclusion that the 4th patient is also having a heart attack before genuinely considering other potential causes. In fact, if some of the findings from the examination don't exactly line up with what they initially think, then they could chalk it up to an "uncommon presentation" of their initial thoughts as opposed to potentially from another cause.

2. *Confirmation bias:* This takes the anchoring bias one step further; the clinician will only check findings that will confirm their initial suspicions, and tend to ignore those that don't support them. If someone presents with a generic symptom like fatigue, one doctor may suspect something like depression so strongly that he doesn't actually consider checking labs or imaging for other conditions. He'll tend to make the story fit the diagnosis of choice, instead of the other way around. If that same person is found to have

lost weight in the last few months as well, then they may use that as justification for their initial theory (they aren't eating because they're depressed) instead of broadening the search to include checking for something like cancer.

3. *Recency bias:* This phenomenon is characterized by what first comes to a physician's mind when creating a list, usually based on what they've recently seen or read about, as opposed to what's the most likely. A doctor who has just finished reading about brain tumors is more likely to jump to a type of brain tumor as a likely diagnosis if someone has presented with headaches for some time, despite the fact that they occur much less frequently than migraines and other causes. They should still include that in the differential diagnosis, but it may not be the first thing they check in the average headache case.

Apart from cognitive bias, the other component of intuitive reasoning involves implicit biases, or how we create cognitive shortcuts when it comes to other people. This is colored by our own personal experiences growing up. Everything from where we grew up, to how our parents raised us, to the people we've been exposed to in our life shapes all of us constantly. The worst part is that we all know about these biases, but that oftentimes alone isn't enough to prevent them.

Luckily, all is not lost. The major way that we combat these biases is by putting tools into place that allow for reflection. During our residency training, our mentors and seniors constantly have us explain our thought processes, and actively reflect on things we may have missed. We also implement "cognitive forcing strategies", where we evaluate a test or lab completely so we avoid missing another potential problem. An x-ray that was obtained to check for pneumonia may also show a rib fracture, but we might miss the latter if the search for abnormalities stops after we locate the pneumonia. As for addressing cognitive biases, more residencies and hospital systems are considering diversity and diverse experiences as a factor in their selection process, which helps not only the patients of that particular demographic but often increases awareness of inequities present in other historically underrepresented groups.

We aim to develop these good cognitive habits early, but will likely miss something at some point, simply because we're human, and we are always limited in resources. So the takeaways from this chapter include:

1. **Ask what is the most likely diagnosis and prognosis (expected course and outcomes).** Your doctor should be open in their thought process about what's the most likely cause of what's going on, but if they aren't then make sure to ask them! Feel free to ask them for the medical term for the condition, and where you can find more information about it. You can also ask what to expect throughout the course of the illness: how long you should expect the symptoms to last, what will happen with and without treatment, how long until treatment takes effect, what side effects may you expect to experience, etc. Especially with conditions that are "clinically diagnosed" (i.e. just based on the history), monitoring the course of the disease may be the only way to "clinically confirm" the disease. If there's a significant amount of variability in what you're experiencing vs what you were told to expect, that alone is a great reason to go back to the doctor for a re-evaluation.

2. **If we don't know what it is, do we know what it's not? What should we be on the lookout for?** If you find yourself back at

the doctor's office with the same complaint, then there's a chance that your doctor's first answer may not have been the right one. Sometimes healthcare is more of a journey than a "one-stop-shop", and you need to make sure that your doctor or other healthcare provider is committed to that journey with you. They should be recognizing their own pitfalls and referring to a specialist when needed. As with any concern (headache, chest pain, shortness of breath, etc), they need to be able to tell you the "red flag" symptoms to watch out for and when you need to go to the ER.

3. **If your doctor isn't listening to you, find one that will!** As a patient, there really isn't much you can address with regard to heuristics and biases. You can't expect perfection since we're all human, but you can expect to find someone who will put forth a good effort in providing you with answers. However, if it comes down to it, don't hesitate to switch doctors if you don't feel like you're being listened to or having your concerns taken seriously. You will ultimately always be your own biggest advocate.

By this point, we (as your doctor) have finally hung our hat on the most likely diagnosis we think it is. After taking a thorough history, examining the different parts of your body, and ordering tests to confirm our suspicions, we have arrived at our final list and adjusted the options accordingly.

So now it's time to treat! Or is it…?

7

To Treat or Not to Treat

The human body is nothing short of remarkable. The treatments we've developed over the last few centuries are definitely notable in their own ways, but even those often work by helping the body to heal itself. If we think of the body as being "at war" when dealing with a foreign invader, like during an infection, then all of the treatments we provide would only constitute as tools, while the real soldiers fighting the battle are the immune cells produced by our bodies. There's a reason why, for the average person, you clear a lot of infections on your own. Whether its the common cold or the touch of food poisoning you may have gotten at your favorite restaurant, our bodies naturally have systems in place to deal with these infections.

In the same way that we had to examine whether or not a certain test would be beneficial to order, we have to ask how beneficial it would be to provide a certain treatment, or in other words consider the risk vs benefit. Everything that truly has a benefit also has a risk depending on its context. We often refer to these as "side effects". If you are found to have a blood clot, you would likely receive a medication we like to call an "anti-thrombolytic", or what some people will refer to as a

37

"blood thinner" or (depending on the dose) a "clot buster". However, if you're also found to be actively bleeding, then we may reconsider using that medication since the nature of the medication's effect will worsen your bleeding. Depending on what's the bigger threat to your health, or based on the other treatment modalities available to us, that will help us determine the direction of our treatment. If you listen to someone who promises something as a "cure-all" that simultaneously has "absolutely no side effects", then you can be sure that it likely doesn't have <u>any</u> effects.

Even something as commonplace as exercise (thought to be beneficial to everyone) can be prohibited in some disease states and contexts. If you've got certain heart conditions, for example, certain kinds of exercise may do you more harm than good. Real risk, real benefit. These are general examples, however; make sure you talk with your doctor if you have questions pertaining to your specific situation.

"My Doctor Didn't Even Give Me Anything!"

This is something we hear commonly, especially in the context of someone who comes to the doctor demanding something for the sake of getting something out of their visit. I've had numerous patients seek an office visit with me with the goal of getting something specific in mind by the end of it. You might have even been one of them, and in some cases, it may have been warranted. However, if you find yourself in an interaction with your doctor that isn't going the way you planned, let's examine what's actually going on.

This gap in expectation typically comes from a misunderstanding about what's going on and/or what treatment regimen is indicated in certain instances. If you come into the doctor's office with an earache demanding antibiotics, it's likely because you assume that your ear pain is due to an ear infection. However, if each visit ended with this "shopping cart medicine", where your doctor blindly complied with your demands just to please you, we would be doing you a huge disservice. Part of our job duties, as mentioned earlier in this book, is to determine what's actually going on. Although your insight definitely carries value, you still deserve a complete and thorough investigation into your ailments. Your ear pain could be from an infection, but it could also be from a ruptured eardrum or a variety of other causes.

Now let's say that your doctor agrees that it's an ear infection, but he still won't give you antibiotics- what gives?! Many times doctors will make specific medical decisions based on guidelines released by certain medical societies. Oftentimes those guidelines are organized as flowcharts, and your provider will follow your case by going through that flowchart to see what the recommended next steps are. For instance, in the case of the ear infection we mentioned earlier, there are different recommendations based on the level of severity of the infection, and even the age of the patient affected, all of which were determined after compiling lots of evidence. If the patient is old enough and if the disease is mild enough, then antibiotics aren't always indicated. We might expect the infection to clear up on its own with minimal risk of complications, or that antibiotics won't give a significant benefit. In that case, you might have been told to just take some Ibuprofen (an anti-inflammatory pain reliever), rest, and avoid getting anything in your ears. This is just one example of many, all to say that there's a complicated balance that we have to assess every time we're presented with a medical dilemma in front of us. Sometimes the answers are clear cut, and other times they aren't.

The decision <u>not</u> to treat is sometimes just as important as the decision to treat. If you get the occasional abdominal pain after eating fatty foods, you might consider changing your diet before immediately undergoing an operation to remove your gallbladder. Even though that's an example of a routine surgery that many undergo, there's always a risk to every procedure, and if you find that your pain isn't that frequent, it may be beneficial to address your lifestyle choices first. In the end, our decision not to treat is best summarized by the phrase we learned in medical school: "First, do no harm".

"My Doctor Just Wants to Push Pills!"

An elderly woman with high blood pressure goes to see her doctor for a check-up. At her last visit, the blood pressure medicine she was placed on previously seemed to do its job; however, today she's found to have high blood pressure again. Confused, you asked her about any recent changes in her life, or any changes in her diet, all of which don't provide any further answers. Finally, you ask her about her blood pressure medicine, to which she replies "Oh, I stopped taking that weeks ago ever since it fixed my blood pressure!"

This phenomenon of "doctors just throwing pills at patients" is the other end of the spectrum we examine with our patients. I find this most commonly stated in the context of treating chronic conditions like diabetes and hypertension. To be honest, this is a fair question to ask- why is it that you might have to take certain medications for certain conditions? And once you have certain diagnoses, are you doomed to take medication for it for the rest of your life? In certain disease states, like a bacterial infection (e.g. pneumonia), most people can agree that an antibiotic course lasting a set number of days would be the most reasonable course of action to pursue. However, once we cross into the land of "chronic illness", certain guidelines may recommend certain treatments, but many times fail to successfully address the root of the problem. If someone develops hypertension after gaining weight, and (importantly!) other kidney ailments have been ruled out, then it could be reasonable to assume that the increased resistance on their arteries could be due to the increased weight they've accumulated. Too many times I've seen doctors prescribe medicine indefinitely, and only give halfhearted advice on losing weight. A more reasonable approach, if it's been determined that your problem is caused by something reversible and in your control, is to create a concrete plan and create the expectation that the medicine will only be required (to decrease mortality, otherwise known as your chance of dying from the disease) so long as the root causes are not addressed.

We also see this often in Type 2 Diabetes, which broadly can be thought of as the body's decreasing sensitivity to insulin, or the hormone produced by the pancreas that's responsible for regulating your blood sugar. It initially starts out with our bodies being flooded with glucose (sugar), which we can largely contribute to the American Diet (at least here in America). With occasional large spikes in glucose, our pancreas will respond by releasing a corresponding level of insulin to signal to the body to make use of whatever glucose is available for energy. If the occasional glucose spikes become *regular* glucose spikes, our bodies eventually form a tolerance to the insulin, and won't respond as strongly as before. If you've ever sat in a building where an alarm was going off for an extended period of time, tolerance here can be thought of as the difference between how you felt at minute 1 vs minute 20. Although it's still annoying at minute 20, your brain doesn't react as vividly as it did at the beginning since it has had some time to get used to it.

The way that diabetes is diagnosed is by checking a lab value called "Hemoglobin A1C", which gives us a picture of your glucose levels over the last 3 months. Simply put, if its value is over 6.5, you are diagnosed with diabetes. If the value is between 5.7 and 6.4, that is classified as "pre-diabetes". In the pre-diabetic stage, the emphasis is typically placed on reversing the disease course and preventing progression to full-blown diabetes. Diet is the most important factor here, but some medications may be introduced to help increase the body's sensitivity (and therefore response) to insulin. However, once the disease becomes severe enough, we typically have to start you on insulin. The tricky part about starting insulin is that now we've introduced a new risk into the equation— the possibility of hypoglycemia, or low blood sugar. And even worse, it often assumes that the disease will stay the same or only continue to get worse, which means you won't get any better! For example, if one patient was started on Insulin because initially her diet alone wasn't enough to control her blood glucose levels, she might run into trouble with low blood sugars if she drastically tries to cut down on her carbs (a common source of glucose) or engages in spontaneous, rigorous exercise (increases the demand for glucose), even though both of which were encouraged in the early stages of diabetes development to control her blood sugars. Therefore, she now has to eat a certain amount of carbs to make sure her glucose levels stay above a certain amount while taking the insulin, something she didn't have to worry about earlier. Increasing her carbs will not improve her diabetes, but it will prevent the complication of hypoglycemia while on insulin, which is managing her diabetes (which here can be thought of as decreasing the chance of further medical complications and death from uncontrolled diabetes). This is a vicious cycle that can be challenging to break, but not impossible. What it requires is a close partnership between patient and doctor (and often diabetes specialists), where if appropriate measures are being taken (including appropriate diet and exercise), the dose of insulin can eventually be lowered and potentially even completely stopped! However, there may be exceptions in certain cases, but it should always be presented as an option whenever possible.

So the question of "To Treat or Not To Treat" is not one that we take lightly. Whether our goals are to decrease the length of time you're sick with something, or whether we're trying to prevent future complications, they always have to be weighed against the risks. Sometimes that risk is an individual side effect, and other times it can be something larger. One of the other major reasons we don't like to throw antibiotics at everything is because of the concept of "antibiotic resistance", or what some describe as accidentally developing a "superbug". The idea here is that if we don't completely kill off the colony of bacteria that's causing a specific disease (which we do by taking the <u>complete</u> course of antibiotics we're prescribed), any bacteria that remain can repopulate and mutate during that process. The more times we give the bacteria a chance to replicate and mutate, the more likely it is that eventually, one day they'll produce a mutation in their DNA that will allow them to resist a certain antibiotic. It's already happened in many cases: one of the first and most common examples is seen in the case of penicillin. Since it was used as a panacea when it was first discovered in 1941, it only took until 1942 for the first penicillin-resistant germ to come about. In the case of methicillin, a cousin of the well-known penicillin, its methicillin-resistant counterpart was discovered the same year as the drug, both of which occurred in 1960. You might know it as MRSA, or Methicillin-resistant Staphylococcus aureus. If you or anyone you know has ever had a MRSA infection, you know that those are incredibly difficult to treat, and everyone who steps in and out of a room of a patient with MRSA is always gowned and gloved for contact precautions to limit its potential spread.

So, what are the takeaway points and questions we want to keep in mind here?

1. What is this medication that you put me on? How does it work? What are some potential side effects I might experience? (Most common? Most concerning?)
2. What will happen if I don't take this medication? Does it affect how well I'll heal or does it just speed up the natural process?
3. How long will I be taking this medication? What determines how long I'll be on this medication? Is there any path forward for me to come off of these medications sometime in the future?
4. What are some concerning signs or symptoms of over or under-treating? At what point should I be concerned enough to come to the hospital?

This list is not all-inclusive, so if anything else comes to mind ask away! These are just some examples of questions that can help with your dialogue, but combined with all of the other ones previously mentioned in this book, hopefully, it'll start to give you a new perspective on healthcare! And with that new perspective, I hope it'll empower you to see the opportunity to take ownership of your health responsibly and place control back in your own hands.

8

"The perfect encounter doesn't exi-"

I f you've made it this far, you've seen how we get through an entire patient encounter, assuming we get the answer right the first time. If you have something a little more complicated, it's not uncommon for you to go through this process multiple times, sometimes with multiple providers and specialists. Is this really how the process is supposed to work? When you have an imperfect system in an imperfect world run by humans (who are imperfect by nature), it's not surprising to see problems. Best-case scenario, you might have to see the doctor more than once; worst-case scenario, someone dies. With stakes as high as these you might think that we, as a society, would prioritize our resources into saving as many lives as possible and preventing as many deaths as possible, but sadly, as with most systemic change, it's not that simple. For instance, it wasn't until someone by the name of Libby Zion passed away in 1984 at the hands of a resident who had been working for 36 hours straight that we finally had laws passed and implemented that limited the number of hours resident physicians could work.

Change historically came at the expense of human lives. Even some-

45

thing as simple as antiseptics in hand-washing, introduced by Ignaz Semmelweis, a Hungarian obstetric physician in the 1840s, was seen as extremely controversial for his time. Not only were many people not fond of trying out his new chlorine-based scrub, as there was no universal understanding about microbes at this time, but many thought that the issue of maternal mortality seen in the clinics at that time was not severe enough to properly investigate, and the disease of "puerperal fever" was ultimately seen as "inevitable". Even when he began to implement his hand-washing techniques and experienced a significant decrease in mortality for the mothers in his ward, that wasn't enough to change everyone's mind. By the end of his life, he had ended up locked away in an asylum, where he was beaten, tortured, and ultimately died 2 weeks later. Although sources vary on the specific cause of death, many believe it was (ironically) from the same infection he had spent his life fighting against.

Luckily, times have largely changed for the better in many ways, but that doesn't mean we don't have a lot we can improve on in today's day and age. The development of insurance companies and hospital systems has complicated health care just as much as they've "helped" it if not more. Up until now, we've talked a lot about how healthcare works on a micro level- that is, solely between the doctor and her patient. To truly get the full picture of the scenario requires an examination of how healthcare works on a macro level: how people gain access to healthcare, how they move through the hospital system, how to make sure the correct problems are addressed without introducing new ones, how insurance companies play a role, and how to make sure we prevent readmission for preventable problems. Each of those concepts is large enough to constitute their own book, which is why they won't be fully addressed today. Some people have put excellent books out there addressing some of these issues already: *To Err Is Human* by the

National Institute of Medicine (explores how medical errors are made with possible solutions), and *Never Pay the First Bill: And Other Ways to Fight the Health Care System and Win* by Marshall Allen (a great resource for individuals stuck with a large healthcare bill) are just a few that immediately come to mind.

Admittedly I have much less experience in the politics of healthcare than I do in the practical application of medicine, but I know enough to tell you that these are issues that cannot be solely addressed by one doctor, and instead will likely require legislation down the line. Not only that but to address some of the largest issues plaguing healthcare, we need to re-imagine how to structure it so it can address what it needs to. According to the Peterson-KFF Health System Tracker, in 2021 the US spent more than double the average of most other wealthy countries per person on healthcare (US: $12,914 vs Average of comparable countries: $6,125), and our outcomes aren't much better for it. In fact, the same tracker showed the US was significantly worse than its peers in long-term health outcomes, which includes measurements like life expectancy, "years of life lost" (a metric that gives more weight to lives lost at younger ages), maternal mortality, and much more. Many people claim that spending a lot of money on healthcare is a positive thing, but if we aren't getting close to the desired outcomes of living healthier lives, then what good is the money we're spending doing? Without knowing where the money we're spending is actually ending up, we won't be addressing the root of the problem.

So, armed with this book, we should be able to address some healthcare issues at least on the micro level mentioned earlier. It's easy to get caught up in all the problems of healthcare, and if we're not careful, we can start to feel hopeless and overwhelmed by all the inequities of the system. However, remembering that there are parts to the equation that we can also control (our own health, our own diet, how much we exercise, our own sense of purpose and connections, etc) can help us take back some power in our lives. Research has shown time and time again that those who take personal responsibility for the situations they find themselves in continually find themselves in better situations. Everyone is capable of having this "internal locus of control", and the more we can remember that, the more we can keep control of our lives.

With this book, I want to empower people to engage with this sense of internal control by teaching them to ask the right questions to their doctors so that they can be actively involved in their own healthcare, instead of just passive observers. Not every doctor you encounter will have the same views on this— I'm sure some physicians who were trained some time ago will prefer to be the sole drivers of the conversation. However, this book is to inform you, the patient, that it doesn't have to be that way. Although the doctor you're talking to may have a deeper understanding of the concepts of medicine, you are the expert on what's happening to you. If you find that someone is trying to explain to you how you're feeling (instead of giving you a possible explanation of what may be happening to you), just know that that could be a form of gaslighting. The times that doctors are explaining away your symptoms prematurely are typically from their own biases, many of which we've covered earlier in this book. Many of those doctors might generally mean well, while the more abrasive ones you might come across are likely burned out by the system they've been serving.

So, as a final summary and teaching point, I'd like to end with some expectations that you deserve to have of your doctor, along with the ones you should have of yourself.

Expectations you should have of your doctor:

1. **Your doctor should listen to what you say and take your complaints seriously.** This has historically been more of a problem for women and people of color, and a lot of it has to do with the history of sexism and racism in medicine. (If you don't believe me, look up the history of the word "hysteria" and the origins of the speculum) Although there have been large improvements compared to even a hundred years ago, in reality, it's only been a few generations since then, so the problems from years ago just look different now. Give your best effort to communicate what's going on and what's concerning you. If you feel like you're being brushed off, a good tactic is to ask, "At what point do I need to be worried about these symptoms?" (how long should I wait to go to the hospital, or what other symptoms might pop up that means my condition has gotten worse? etc) And if all of that doesn't seem to work, feel free to switch providers!

2. **They should address (at least one) complaint as fully as possible.** If your complaint is not addressed fully, it could be the case that it's a more complicated case than was anticipated so it's not uncommon for you to have to follow up with several visits to monitor the condition. At the same time, please don't try to unload all of your problems and expect them all to get fixed. If you do have a list of concerns bothering you, mentioning that at the beginning can help you and your doctor create a plan to manage them.

3. **They should take any and all questions you have about your own health.** You should feel safe while talking to your doctor about any health concerns. Time constraints, like what was mentioned earlier in this very book, can sometimes throw a wrench in our plans, but there should be open communication as best as possible. If your doctor makes you feel generally unwelcome to ask questions, that is a red flag. You should feel empowered about

taking control of your own health, and your doctor should be a great resource for you to take advantage of. On the other hand, outside of your appointment time, don't expect an immediate response to your medical question if you contact your doctor's office. Many offices have online portals that allow patients to send questions to their doctors, and many doctor offices have policies that allow for at least 24 or even up to 72 hours for the doctor to respond. It's not vindictive, it's simply a matter of providing the doctor the flexibility to respond whenever they can given the unpredictability of their schedules along with their immense workload and constant deadlines for their tasks and notes. Familiarize yourself with the policy of your personal doctor's office to make the most use of this.

Expectations you should have of You, the Patient:

1. **You need to be the one who cares the most about your own health.** In a perfect world, that would be closely followed by your support system of family and friends, followed closely after that by your doctor. Most of us care very much about our patients, but we can't carry you along on your health journey for you; we can only walk with you and show you the way to go. We don't have the resources to come to your house and pull you off the couch to encourage you to go for that run. Our time is already severely limited managing all of the patients we have, so you have to do your part and meet us halfway. But if there is a specific way that we can support you, be sure to let us know!

2. **Tell the truth, the whole truth, and nothing but the truth.** Sometimes it might feel embarrassing to bring up certain topics or answer certain questions, but your doctor should be creating

a judgment-free zone. Our main priority is you, and anything you can tell us that'll help us help you is extremely important. Don't make us play detective if we don't have to, the only person you'll harm is yourself. The other major reason patients may lie to their doctors is to prevent themselves from feeling shame and their doctors from feeling disappointed if they haven't met their personal goals. Although we'll support you whenever you hit your milestones, we won't judge you if you don't because we recognize it's hard. I would rather you come clean with your updates (still having trouble losing weight, eating healthy, stopping smoking, etc) instead of lying and saying you've got everything together because the former will transform the conversation into one that can address potential barriers, while the latter will keep the two of us stuck with the same problem. If we want to get ahead of any major problems, we need to make honesty a priority.

3. **Please be patient.** As you've learned throughout this book, there are many potential problems that can arise in healthcare that can delay your office visit. Even the most prepared provider is bound to experience surprises. Bringing a book ahead of time (like this one!) or practicing meditation are great ways to expand the mind and take advantage of the stillness of your exam room.

And that's it! Manage these expectations and you'll be well on your way to getting the most out of your visit.

9

Conclusion

If you've gotten to the end of this book, congratulations! Hopefully, it allowed you to examine a new perspective that you may not have been aware of before. It's easy to classify an entire system as "broken" and "complicated" and leave it at that, but for there to be real change in the world there has to be enough people who are aware of the problem's existence, and a large enough proportion of those people to care enough to do something about it. Just because something can't be perfectly fixed doesn't mean that we can't try our best to make it a little better. This book by itself is a far cry from significantly meaningful change, but if it can plant some seeds for conversation in the future then I believe it will have done a meaningful job. If healthcare encounters were just limited to the patient-doctor relationship, then solutions would be much easier to reach. However, a notable behemoth that requires its own book to cover, like I mentioned before, is that of the insurance companies. That topic alone would require much more time, energy, and research to completely investigate, so I decided not to touch on it much in this book. At some point in the future, that may be a topic I investigate.

However, if you enjoyed reading this book as much as I enjoyed writing it, or if you learned anything new, consider leaving a nice review on Amazon! That would be much appreciated and it would let me know if I should write another book like this in the future. :)

In summary, the point of this book is to put a little more power back in the hands of you, the patient. True healthcare is built on patient autonomy, where you as the patient have all the understanding about your condition to make truly informed decisions about your own care. Our job is to discern what the situation is and provide you with all of the information we have available, along with our recommendation on the course of treatment. Your job is to be present and digest the information we've presented to you, and then translate that into what you want for yourself and your future based on your values. Most times it'll be easy: taking antibiotics for the occasional infection typically has much more benefit than risk. However, some people find themselves in more troubling, not-so-clear-cut cases. If you happen to be newly diagnosed with Stage IV terminal colon cancer, do you suffer through surgery, chemo, and/or radiation to potentially give you a few more years but with less quality of life, or do you prioritize your quality of life and make the best out of the time you have left? This is a simplistic example but one that is meant to illustrate that sometimes there is no one right answer, just your answer. We will always provide all available options and let you decide. Often some people may ask their physicians "If you were me, what would you do?" Depending on who you're talking to, you may or may not get an answer to that question. So the last call to action I have for you is this: Know yourself. Learn what matters to you in life, and what it means to have a meaningful life for you. In the modern day of constant distractions, it's easier than ever to miss your own life. And, as Socrates said himself, "The unexamined life is not worth living".

References

Summerton N. (2008). The medical history as a diagnostic technology. *The British journal of general practice : the journal of the Royal College of General Practitioners, 58*(549), 273–276. https://doi.org/10.3399/bjgp08X279779

Facts about Down Syndrome | CDC. (2023, October 10). Centers for Disease Control and Prevention. https://www.cdc.gov/ncbddd/birth defects/downsyndrome.html

Lumbreras, B., Donat, L., & Hernández-Aguado, I. (2010). Incidental findings in imaging diagnostic tests: a systematic review. *The British journal of radiology, 83*(988), 276–289. https://doi.org/10.1259/bjr/98067945

Beigelman-Aubry, C., Hill, C., & Grenier, P. A. (2007). Management of an incidentally discovered pulmonary nodule. *European radiology, 17*(2), 449–466. https://doi.org/10.1007/s00330-006-0399-7

History.com Editors. (2009, November 24). *German scientist discovers x-rays.* HISTORY. Retrieved October 26, 2023, from https://www.history.com/this-day-in-history/german-scientist-discovers-x-rays

Imaging, C. (2022, July 25). *History of the CT scan.* Mobile CT Rental - Mobile Imaging Rental and Lease. https://catalinaimaging.com/histor

y-ct-scan/

Garet, L. (2020, December 26). *History of MRIs and the Evolution of This Life-Saving Technology.* Ezra. Retrieved October 26, 2023, from https://ezra.com/blog/history-of-mri-scans

Choby, B. A. (2009b, March 1). *Diagnosis and Treatment of Streptococcal Pharyngitis.* AAFP. Retrieved October 26, 2023, from https://www.a afp.org/pubs/afp/issues/2009/0301/p383.html#treatment-of-gabhs-pharyngitis

CDC. (2024, June 27). *Rheumatic Fever: All You Need to Know | CDC.* Retrieved October 26, 2023, from https://www.cdc.gov/groupastrep/diseases-public/rheumatic-fever.html

Lenco Diagnostic Laboratory. (2020, September 27). *The Brief History of Phlebotomy: Why and When People First Start Blood Drawn | Blog | www.lencolab.com.* www.lencolab.com. Retrieved October 26, 2023, from https://www.lencolab.com/publications/2020/9/the-brief-hist ory-of-phlebotomy.html

Whelehan, D. F., Conlon, K. C., & Ridgway, P. F. (2020). Medicine and heuristics: cognitive biases and medical decision-making. *Irish journal of medical science, 189*(4), 1477–1484. https://doi.org/10.1007/s11845-020-02235-1

Balakrishnan, K., & Arjmand, E. M. (2019). The Impact of Cognitive and Implicit Bias on Patient Safety and Quality. *Otolaryngologic clinics of North America, 52*(1), 35–46. https://doi.org/10.1016/j.otc.2018.08.016

American Medical Association, & Smith, T. (2021, February 4). *4 widespread cognitive biases and how doctors can overcome them.* American Medical Association. Retrieved October 26, 2023, from https://www.ama-assn.org/delivering-care/ethics/4-widespread-cognitive-biases-and-how-doctors-can-overcome-them

Institute of Medicine (US) Committee on Quality of Health Care in America; Kohn LT, Corrigan JM, Donaldson MS, editors. To Err is Human: Building a Safer Health System. Washington (DC): National Academies Press (US); 2000. Available from: https://www.ncbi.nlm.nih.gov/books/NBK225182/

Doherty, T. S., & Carroll, A. E. (2020, September 1). *Believing in Overcoming Cognitive Biases.* AMA Journal of Ethics. https://doi.org/10.1001/amajethics.2020.773

Ramakrishnan, K. (2007, December 1). *Diagnosis and Treatment of Otitis Media.* AAFP. Retrieved October 26, 2023, from https://www.aafp.org/pubs/afp/issues/2007/1201/p1650.html

Drew, C. (2023b, October 21). *22 Heuristics Examples (The Types of Heuristics).* Helpful Professor. Retrieved October 26, 2023, from https://helpfulprofessor.com/heuristics-examples-types/

Marewski, J. N., & Gigerenzer, G. (2012). Heuristic decision making in medicine. *Dialogues in clinical neuroscience, 14*(1), 77–89. https://doi.org/10.31887/DCNS.2012.14.1/jmarewski

Hughes, T. M., Dossett, L. A., Hawley, S. T., & Telem, D. A. (2020). Recognizing heuristics and bias in clinical decision-making. *Annals of Surgery, 271*(5), 813–814. https://doi.org/10.1097/sla.0000000000003699

Stanford Lifestyle Medicine. (n.d.). *Stanford Lifestyle Medicine Pillars of Health*. Lifestyle Medicine. Retrieved October 26, 2023, from https://longevity.stanford.edu/lifestyle/lifestyle-pillars/

CDC. (2022, October 5). *How Antimicrobial Resistance Happens*. www.CDC.gov. Retrieved October 26, 2023, from https://www.cdc.gov/drugresistance/about/how-resistance-happens.html

Patient Safety Network. (2019, September 7). *Duty Hours and Patient Safety*. PSNet.ahrq.gov. Retrieved October 26, 2023, from https://psnet.ahrq.gov/primer/duty-hours-and-patient-safety

Zoltán, I. (2023, September 12). Ignaz Semmelweis. Encyclopedia Britannica. https://www.britannica.com/biography/Ignaz-Semmelweis

Lopez-Garrido, G. (2023, August 14). Locus of Control Theory In Psychology: Definition & Examples. *Simply Psychology*. Retrieved October 26, 2023, from https://www.simplypsychology.org/locus-of-control.html

Famakinwa, J. (2012). IS THE UNEXAMINED LIFE WORTH LIVING OR NOT? *Think, 11*(31), 97-103. doi:10.1017/S1477175612000073 https://www.cambridge.org/core/journals/think/article/abs/is-the-unexamined-life-worth-living-or-not/8D5EC7FCA494A8B9A5E5D02BADAB6182

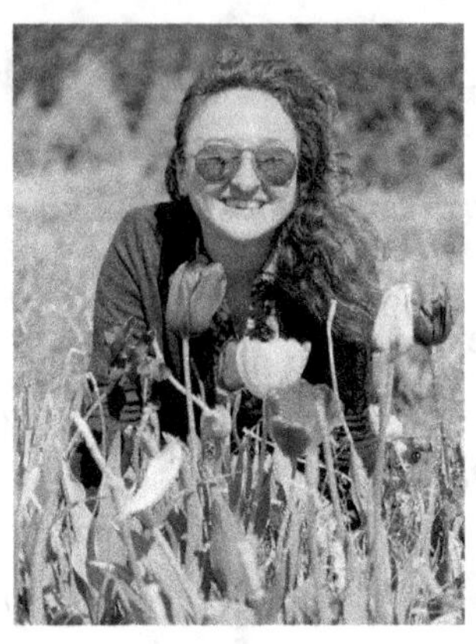

About the Author

Dr. Justyna Szymonik was born in a small town in Poland but was raised outside of Atlanta, Georgia for most of her life. This book was based on her experiences in medical school as well as her time in Family Medicine residency. She loves chocolate, ballroom dancing, and her black cat named Tuki. This is her first book but she is looking forward to writing more!